Smoking

Donna Kakonge was born in Kitchener, Waterloo, Canada and grew up in Toronto. At the age of 14 she started to smoke cigarettes to look cool for an older boy she had a crush on. This book is about the stories of those people who have successfully conquered the urge to smoke.

Kakonge is also the author of *What Happened to the Afro?*, *How to Write Creative Non-fiction*, *Spiderwoman*, *Morning English Lessons*, *In My Pocket*, editor of *Being Healthy: Selected Works from the Internet*, writer of *Do Not Know*, *My Story of Transportation*, *Draft*:

eSpirituality Chats, reporter and producer of a CD of radio documentaries called "Nine," writer of *Journalism Stories Collection, Digital Journals and Numerology, Where I Was, Draft: Part Two, Radio and Television Announcing, Ugandan Travelogue* and narrated two audio stories from *Spiderwoman*; "Matoke" and "Church Sunday." The latter appeared in *Headlight Anthology*. *School Works* is a collection of essays written at the undergraduate and graduate level. *Yes, School Works* are all communications essays written while she did graduate work in Montreal with Concordia University. *School Works – Other Essays* are from undergraduate work done at Carleton University in Ottawa, Canada. *The Best of Donna Magazine* highlights her online magazine which can be viewed at: http://kakonged.wordpress.com. *Old Romance* is Kakonge's 32nd book. It is a book of short stories about old romances. *How to Start Your Own Teaching and Writing Business* is Kakonge's most recent book. Donna Kakonge lives in Toronto, Canada.

www.donnakakonge.com

BOOKS AND CDS BY DONNA KAKONGE

What Happened to the Afro?

How to Write Creative Non-fiction

Spiderwoman

My Roxanne

Being Healthy: Selected Works from the Internet (edited)

Do Not Know

My Story of Transportation

Draft: eSpirituality Chats

"Nine" (CD)

Journalism Stories Collection

School Works – Other Essays

Honest Psychic Chats

The Write Heart

Listening to Music

This is How the Egyptians Fell

Natural Beauty

Random Bibliography of Media Books and Internet
Resources

My Mind Book

Stories in Red and Yellow: Digging up Work Done in
Yesteryear

The Best of Donna Magazine

Dropouts

Old Romance

How to Start Your Own Teaching and Writing Business

Smoking

Donna Kakonge

Lulu.com

FIRST EDITION LULU INTERNATIONAL EDITION,

January 2010

Copyright 2010 by Donna Kay Kakonge, M.A.

All rights researched under International and Pan-American Copyright Conventions. Published in the United States by Lulu.com.

Library and Archives of Canada Cataloguing in Publication Data

Kakonge, Donna Kay Cindy
Smoking
ISBN:

Book Design by Dreamstime.com

Manufactured in the United States.

Conversation: Stopping Smoking is Easy

I have been trying to stop again for months. Ever since the coldest winter to hit Toronto in decades fell in 2008. This is also the year of the rat...the year that is supposed to be my year, as well as the year of all other rats out there. It is also the year I turn 36 where smoking to be cool does not become funny anymore. My health is at risk here. I had always heard growing up that a woman should not smoke over the age of 35.

So, I went outside armed with my pack of DuMaurier king size and sat in a regular spot with a cigarette dangling from my mouth. My neighbour next door who is inspiring in the sense that he plays all kinds of sports and is a health "nut" makes me look really bad when he is always driving off for rugby practice and I am just sitting there smoking. My life could slip away just sitting in different chairs outside my apartment that my Dad finds while doing his paper delivery and smoking away.

I let Devin know what I was doing. He wished me luck. As soon as his car drove off, I started to smoke. It felt regular, it felt like it always does.

By time my neighbour Cheryl came along rolling a cart to take back to the neighbourhood Loblaws, I told her what I was doing too. I was thankful she is a nurse so if anything happened to me, she could help.

I could not get past four cigarettes, even that fourth one was hard. I could feel the bile rising in my throat the minute I got back into my apartment. My cheeks kept getting bigger as it housed the bile that I was determined not to let spill onto my newly swept wood floors. I opened the bathroom and spit into the toilet. Using my socked foot, I cleaned up the vomit that spilled onto the floor. I was sick...I accomplished what I wanted.

I left the bathroom and was moving to put my coat and scarf back in their proper place when another round of sickness hit me. Back to the toilet, again with the sock.

This time it was more satisfying because I was sure I would not smoke again.

I put my things away, threw away the two packs of cigarettes and the four left in the third pack that I had, plus deposited my butts in my Dad's wastebin outside his house next door to mine.

"I smoked myself sick," I told my Dad.

He laughed while drinking a beer and smoking.

"That should last at least three years," I said. "More if I am not stupid enough to start again."

As I went inside my apartment, I said, "I won't smoke again," remembering what Lee (one of my online coaches) told me about the self-fulfilling prophecy. I do believe in that.

As I write this, there is an uncomfortable feeling in my stomach. I feel a little woozy. I am drinking some root beer, since I do not drink. This has been the last bastion of sins I have been trying to eradicate from life. I do not even drink coffee anymore. God grant me with the grace to keep thinking stopping smoking is easy.

Chapter 2

Just had an interview today with someone named Kevin Fairweather for a story I am doing for Canadian Builders Quarterly. Wow, did he ever say something wise he heard someone else say.

"You wake up in the morning aiming for perfection. At the end of the day, you get reality."

So true. I have smoked today. Well, at least I guess it's something legal such as cigarettes. I get scared to think of the day when they may become illegal. What would I do? I would just have to quit and it would be so hard. I really wish I had just not ever started in the first place. I guess everyone has their cross to bear.

Chapter 3

I went back on Kasamba, now known as LivePerson and asked one of the psychics about how I could stop smoking. The person suggested that I put a spoon of lime juice in water and drink it in the morning and evening. They also suggested that I breathe deeply about 10 to 20 times a day, meditate and do yoga. I think these are all good suggestions and I have been trying to implement them. It's May 18, 2008 and I am still smoking, however I am still working on it.

Today I have not been smoking as much. I find the suggestion does help somewhat. I do have faith in all of this. I did some yoga last night with a VHS tape and I hope to get through the whole tape today. I will be back in shape in time enough – I have faith in that. I know yoga and meditation is a really good thing. I have had a doctor I went to a number of months ago and my psychiatrist tells me the same thing.

The day is not over yet – neither are my efforts to stop smoking.

Chapter 3

This brings us to present day. Wednesday, January 13, 2010 an
am still smoking. I'm OK with it. I am not trying to make mys
sick anymore. I'm focusing on my goals and dreams and worki
hard. I can still be a good person even if I do smoke. God think
I'm perfect any way. God thinks we are all perfect.

Here are some really special people that rose and conquered the
challenge of quitting smoking. Read on…

Chapter 4

Deb Bailey is CEO of Power Women Magazine and Radio Show.

Bailey quit smoking 10 years ago using the cold turkey method. She owns a power women magazine and radio show. She started at the age of 14 after being dared by her friends.

"I quit cold turkey and went through HELL, but so glad I quit," says Bailey. "I had withdrawals, panic attacks, night sweats, muscles drew under chin, nightmares, you name it."

She tells teens and others around her not to start. She has come hate it.

Dr. Nancy Irwin is a psychotherapist, clinical hypnotist, author speaker. She quit smoking nearly 13 years ago after having smoked for 20 to 25 years. She now makes a living helping othe to do the same with therapeutic hypnosis. She has a 90 per cent success rate.

Irwin is a doctor of psychology and author of *You-Turn: Changing Direction in Midlife* (available on Amazon.com).

She started smoking at 18.

"At age 42 by following professional's advice: pick a date in advance, get psychologically geared up for it, and then throw away all your leftovers and ashtrays, and clean the house and car! Set up activities to distract yourself and know that you are stronger than the urge."

Irwin believes that it is social influence that causes many teens to fall prey to smoking. They are not deliberately smoking to flush 4,000 toxins through their systems, rather they are trying to be cool, fit in, look older/sexy/macho/"bad"/tough, flaunt authority, etc.

"When they realize there are 100's of ways to get those needs met without poison, they can be free."

Irwin says, at birth you were given one body to last your entire life, and with it the choice to make it the best it can be…or not.

Nancy Irwin is based in Los Angeles, California and her website is: www.drnancyirwin.com.

PW Mooney used to smoke three packs a day. He refers to himself as "Just Joe Smoker," when asked about his credentials.

He started smoking in junior college around 19 years old.

When did he stop smoking?

"Stopped on May 3rd, 1983 [with] baking soda. Truly. A teaspoon of powder baking soda filled by a glass of water (NOT baking soda in the water). Supposedly the baking soda absorbs the nicotine the same it absorbs odours in the refrigerator. After two or three weeks I no longer had the "immediate" urge and was able to mentally stop myself. To this day I still smell the "attraction" when I smell smoke and re-enforce it by saying that it is stupid to smoke."

Mooney has not had a cigarette since. He quit when he was

challenged by Peter Ueberoth, president of the 1984 Olympics, where he worked.

"It was the pre-Olympic water polo event and he caught me smoking. I put a pack of Marlboros [in] an ashtray and book of matches on the coffee table in front of my lounge chair. Kept it there for one year. Could have lit up any time."

PW Mooney lives in Torrence, California.

Ryan Elliott is a hypnoanalyst at The Lightheart Center, as well as an author. He has appeared on the *Oprah* to discuss his book. His book is called *The Secrets from Your Subconscious Mind*.

"I quite smoking 30 some years ago cold turkey," says Elliott. "For the last 25 plus years, I've been treating smokers with hypnoanalysis and obtaining about 85 per cent success over the long term by using two secret techniques."

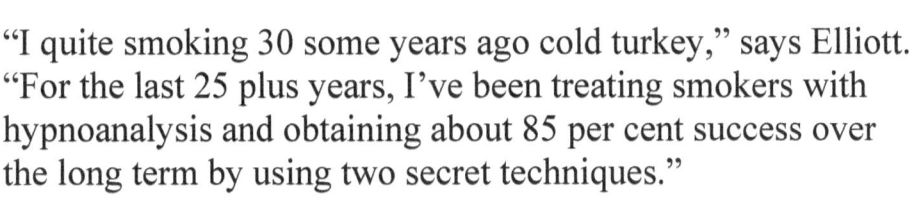

Elliott is a board certified medical hypnoanalyst, author of *The Secrets from Your Subconscious Mind* which can be had at: www.thelightheartcenter.org. There is a very good chapter in the book on smoking. You can click on the "Free Secrets" book page.

He started smoking at the age of 12 in 1960 with the other hoods at the coffee shop near where he grew up. He stopped at age 24, cold turkey, and used a pacifier in his mouth when he had the craving and toothpicks in public.

Elliott says smoking is self destructive, nasty and crapping on other people who smell the smoke.

If you live in the Winfield, Illinois area and would like Ryan Elliott's services, you can contact him on his website at www.thelightheartcenter.org. His email is: seelight@juno.com.

Jim Gerdeman is an author who was a smoker and has now quit. He was fortunate to marry a non-smoking advocate.

"I did quit smoking," says Gerdeman. "I have written a book, *Smoke Signals You too Can Quit*. I have family and friends who have been addicted. Their stories as well as my own offer solutions to stop."

Gerdeman's website has more information at: www.JDGerdeman.com.

Gerdeman says he stopped smoking just before a major business review he had to present. It was not a good time to do it, but he persevered.

"I say it might have cost me my career.

"Society once thought smoking represented health, wealth and success but found it now represents failure, addiction and death. I know many who need to stop but don't, want to stop but can't find the strength. It is bad for us in so many ways."

Gerdeman says he encourages readers to stop smoking the signals from developing the habit and life gripping addiction to nicotine.

Gerdeman lives in Coral Springs, Florida. His email is: JDGerdeman@aol.com.

John Wilder is an author who quit cold turkey. He went to

nursing school as well as attended grad school for clinical psychology and has an undergrad in behavioural science. He started smoking in 1969. He stopped smoking in 1985. He says smoking is dangerous.

Jennifer McDonell is director of Sovereign Clipper, as well as an author. She works with clients to help them quit cigarettes in 60 minutes, guaranteed.

The method used is hypnosis NLP EFT TFT. McDonell started smoking at 24. She quit at 40 after a major change of values. Sometimes she will have a cigarette with a special friend.

"It can be fun," she says.

McDonell says there is always a reason for why someone smokes, such as a negative emotion always drives the need.

She adds it is possible for anyone to quit.

"I have clients who have smoked for 40 years and stopped in ONE session. This work makes it easy for someone to do what they want to do. Even with a guarantee, some people don't decide to stop."

Lorraine Morgan Scott is an author who has successfully quite for 10 years now. She started when she was 12-years-old. She quit smoking on September 9, 1999 at 3:33 p.m.

"First, I knew the time had come that I really wanted to quit. My reason for this was not my health, not money, and not social pressure. It was because my then 4-year-old said, "look mom, I'm 'smoking!" as he imitated putting his fingers to his lips with an invisible cigarette. Second, I purchased the nicotine patch. When I craved a cigarette I would press the patch, smack the patch, or pound the patch. I would mentally envision the nicotine entering my blood stream and running its course. I was on the patch for six to nine weeks (can't remember.) My husband, who was so happy I was no longer smoking, offered the patch for the rest of my life if I wanted it. While wearing the patch, and during those first few weeks, I altered my habits (and my family's) so we didn't linger over meals, didn't go to places where I'd be around smokers, and I didn't drink any alcohol.

Scott adds:

I enjoyed smoking completely. After quitting, maybe 6 years later, I was in the shower and thought how good the cigarette was going to be when I got out - and then realized I'd quit. I didn't like the smoke though. I didn't like mine (I smoked outside, or when in the car - the windows were down.) I didn't like other's smoke, and I couldn't eat around people when they were smoking. But I enjoyed the sensation of the nicotine going through my system.

Scott adds:

I am so glad I quit. I recently celebrated my 10th non-smoking year. I see others who smoke - especially young people, and I feel for them. Neither of my adult children smoke (or ever have) so that is a blessing, and I hope my son never starts. Every once in a while I miss the sensation – not the act or the smell. Not long ago I dreamt I started smoking again and I woke up crying. I do not want to smoke.

Thank you

Thank you to all of you who have taken the time to inspire me and help me create these stories. Most of all...thanks to the readers.

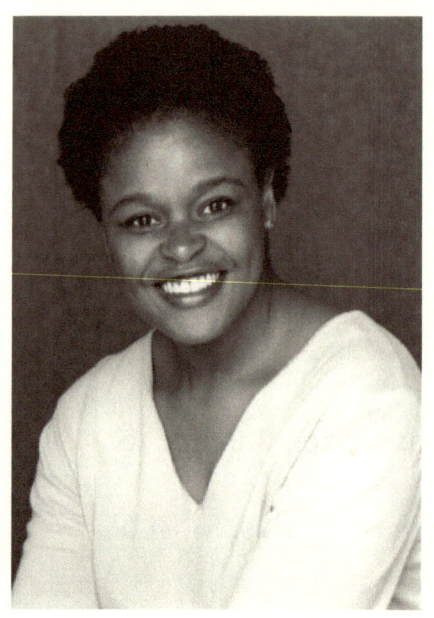

Donna Kakonge (BJ Carleton, MA Concordia) is a

freelance educator, writer and broadcaster teaching

journalism and communications in Toronto, Canada. She's

also taught abroad. She received a Gemini nomination for

work done with the Discovery Channel. Please find out

more information by using the Google search engine below.

Donna's résumé is also available for potential clients.

You can purchase her e-books *what Happened to the Afro?* ,
How to Write Creative Non-fiction, and *Spiderwoman* at her lulu.com storefront. My books are also available on Amazon's Kindle.

She's worked in every form of media, from print, radio, television and online with such places as *the Toronto Star, New Dreamhomes and Condominiums Magazine,* the CBC, BBC, Young People's Press, One80 Youth Media Group and Vision TV. Her work and travel have taken her to such places as Belgium, Germany, Spain, Uganda and South Africa.

Check out the recent stories and audio files for exciting free information.

To contact Donna Kakonge, you can email her at: dkakonge@sympatico.ca.

Also By Donna Kakonge:

What Happened to the Afro?

This graduate research paper is a case study that sheds light on the politics of black hair.

How to Write Creative Non-fiction

Writing is one of the hardest jobs in the world, and this book will give you the help you need to crack the market. Everything you wanted to know about the writing business and how to write, with exercises included.

Spiderwoman

This book of short stories crafted over many years and originally developed in a writing workshop at Carleton University includes the experiences of a young black woman in Canada, experiencing everything from travel to family tragedy and love.

My Roxanne

Written at the age of 17 and revised later in life, this novel is the story of Roxanne and Lance – an interracial couple who go through their ups and downs.

Being Healthy: Selected Works from the Internet

This book is a compilation of works from the Internet related to health that have been edited by Donna Kakonge.

Do Not Know

This book is a collection of literary explorations of madness. A young black woman experiences the challenges and adventures of mental illness.

My Story of Transportation

This book is a memoir of Donna Kakonge's transportation experiences. Everything from roller skates to Jaguars; this is a story of how she has managed to get around.

Draft: Spirituality Chats

On a desperate search for a PhD, Donna Kakonge actually produces doctorate-level work by discovering there is more knowledge in one's common sense than meets the third eye of psychics.

Journalism Stories Collection

From newspapers and magazines such as NuBeing International, Panache, Pride, Share and the Toronto Star

– Donna Kakonge creates a collection of her journalistic stories that span five years of her writing career.

The Education Generation

Perfect for professors, students and anyone in the college or university system in North America, this book has articles and columns that explore the notion of the education generation.

Digital Journals and Numerology

This book is meant to emphasize how powerful keeping a journal can be with the aid of numerology. I started writing one at the age of seven and keeping a journal has been a constant for me – more than some friends, some jobs and some family members. I used to get a thrill selecting my journals to write in. Now I have decided to try something new by using the computer that I already spend so much time on and money on to show how powerful keeping any journal...even a digital journal can be. Using the principles of numerology can also help in chronicling your life.

Other Work:

"Nine"

This is a selection of some of Donna Kakonge's radio documentaries done with the Canadian Broadcasting Corporation, as well as Radio Canada International.

"Matoke"

This audio book brings the story of Matoke from the book Spiderwoman to your ears.

"Church Sunday"

From the book Spiderwoman, an audio story of the story
"Church Sunday," first published in Concordia
University's *Headlight Anthology* and reviewed by the
Montreal Gazette.

In My Pocket

This book was written to help you during the perilous
times we live in.

Morning English Lessons

This is a book that is ideal for helping you hone your

English skills.

Where I Was

This is a memoir of Donna Kakonge's sometimes-difficult life spent in Montreal and her move to the place she grew up in, Toronto.

Draft: Part Two

What happens when you turn to psychics for answers? You discover God.

Radio and Television Announcing

This book gives some fundamental knowledge to radio and television announcing.

Ugandan Travelogue

Donna Kakonge goes back to one of her homelands to discover where home really is.

School Works

A collection of essays Donna Kakonge has done about the black press, black journalists and ethics in filmmaking through undergraduate work at Carleton University in Ottawa, Canada and graduate work at Concordia University in Montreal, Quebec.

Yes, School Works

A collection of communication essays done at the graduate level at Concordia University in Montreal, Canada.

School Works – Other Essays

This is a collection of undergraduate arts essays done at Carleton University in Ottawa, Canada.

Honest Psychic Chats

This conversation with psychics is the last book in the series of psychic chat sessions online.

The Write Heart

This is the last in a series of books about journalism that started with How to Write Creative Non-fiction and followed with Radio and Television Announcing. This book deals with journalistic and non-fiction writing.

Story Ideas: Help For Writer's Block

This is a collection of unfinished stories that writers could pick up on to develop full-length stories.

Listening to Music

The experience of listening to Erykah Badu, Sting and India.Arie.

This is How the Egyptians Fell

Further conversations with psychics lead to a deeper understanding of how bogus this business really is. This is why the Egyptians fell.

Natural Beauty

Tips, information and advice on all forms of being a natural beauty.

Random Bibliography of Media Books and Internet Resources

This is a resource guide for media professionals, as well as students. It is also available as a free download.

My Mind Book

This is a guide of how to manifest the law of attraction.

Stories in Red and Yellow

This is a collection of fiction and non-fiction work.